THE ULTIMATE ENDOMETRIOSIS DIET COOKBOOK

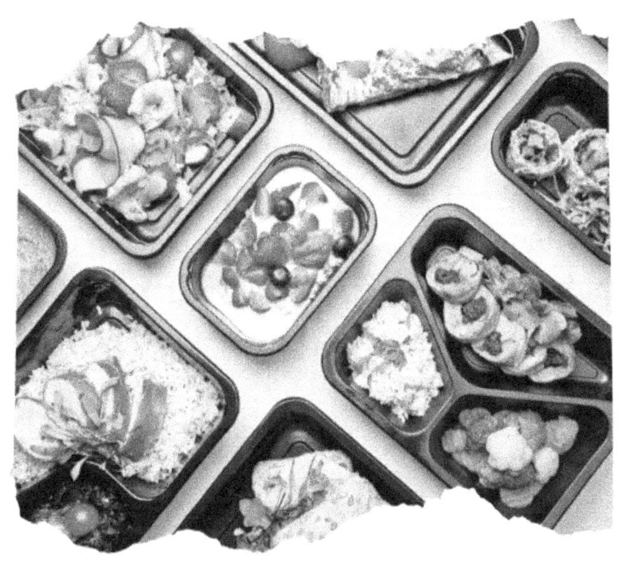

Quick And Easy Nourishing Recipes For Managing Endometriosis And Improve Your Shape To Feel Healthy Again

AMADA L. HEATH

HOW TO USE THIS COOKBOOK

Familiarize Yourself:
Begin by reading through the Endometriosis Diet cookbook thoroughly. Understand the principles behind the recommended dietary guidelines, paying attention to foods that promote anti-inflammatory responses and hormonal balance.

Create a Meal Plan:
Utilize the cookbook's recipes to create a personalized meal plan. Consider factors like taste preferences, dietary restrictions, and individual responses to specific ingredients. A well-planned meal schedule ensures a balanced and nourishing approach.

Compile a Shopping List:
Review each recipe and compile a comprehensive shopping list with the required ingredients. This step simplifies the grocery shopping process and ensures you

have all necessary items on hand when preparing meals.

Meal Preparation:

Set aside dedicated time for meal preparation. Batch-cook elements that can be used across multiple recipes, making the cooking process more efficient during busy days. Following the cookbook's instructions, prepare meals in advance for convenience.

Listen to Your Body:

As you embark on the Endometriosis Diet, pay close attention to how your body responds. Monitor any changes in symptoms, energy levels, and overall well-being. Be open to adjustments, tailoring the cookbook's recommendations to your unique needs for optimal health.

TABLE OF CONTENT

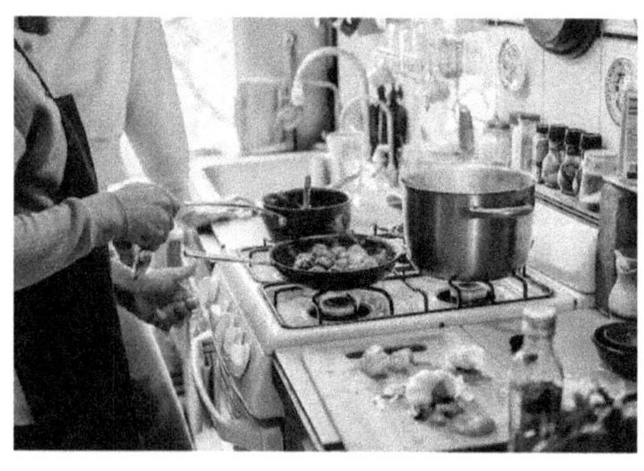

INTRODUCTION

In the small town of Meadowridge, there lived a resilient old woman named Eleanor. At 70 years old, Eleanor had faced numerous challenges in her life, but none as persistent and painful as endometriosis. However, she refused to let this condition dictate her life.

Eleanor had spent years trying different medications and treatments, but none seemed to provide long-lasting relief. It wasn't until she stumbled upon an Endometriosis Diet Cookbook that things began to change. Intrigued by the possibility of managing her symptoms through nutrition, Eleanor decided to give it a try.

The cookbook, written by a nutritionist who had also battled endometriosis, offered a comprehensive guide to foods that could alleviate inflammation and hormonal imbalances associated with the condition.

Eleanor, armed with newfound knowledge, eagerly embraced the challenge of transforming her diet.

She started incorporating more anti-inflammatory foods into her meals, such as leafy greens, fatty fish, and berries. The cookbook emphasized the importance of cutting out inflammatory triggers like gluten and dairy, so Eleanor bid farewell to her beloved pastries and creamy dishes.

Initially, the transition was challenging, but Eleanor was determined. She spent hours in her cozy kitchen, experimenting with recipes from the cookbook, adapting them to suit her taste and preferences. Her culinary skills improved, and she found joy in creating delicious, endometriosis-friendly meals.

As weeks turned into months, Eleanor noticed a significant reduction in her symptoms. The chronic pain that had once plagued her began to subside, and her energy levels increased. Encouraged by these positive changes, Eleanor became an advocate for the endometriosis diet within her community.

She organized weekly gatherings at her home, inviting other women battling endometriosis to share their experiences and exchange recipes. Together, they formed a support network that extended beyond the kitchen, providing emotional support and understanding.

Eleanor's kitchen became a hub of empowerment and resilience, where women discovered the transformative power of mindful eating. The Endometriosis Diet Cookbook became their shared guide, and the town of Meadowridge witnessed a collective shift towards healthier living.

Word of Eleanor's success spread beyond Meadowridge, reaching the author of the cookbook herself. Impressed by Eleanor's dedication and the positive impact she had on her community, the author paid a visit to meet the woman who had turned her words into a beacon of hope.

The encounter was heartwarming, as Eleanor and the cookbook author bonded over shared experiences and a common goal – empowering women to take control of their health. Together, they continued to inspire countless others to embrace the healing power of a well-balanced, endometriosis-friendly diet.

And so, in the small town of Meadowridge, Eleanor's kitchen continued to be a place of transformation, where the aroma of wholesome meals became synonymous with strength, resilience, and the triumph over adversity.

CHAPTER 1: WHAT IS ENDOMETRIOSIS DIET

The Endometriosis Diet, as outlined in the Endometriosis Diet Cookbook, is a targeted nutritional approach designed to alleviate symptoms associated with endometriosis. Endometriosis is a condition where tissue similar to the lining of the uterus grows outside the uterus, causing inflammation, pain, and hormonal imbalances. The diet focuses on reducing inflammation, balancing hormones, and supporting overall health.

The cookbook emphasizes the importance of anti-inflammatory foods. Leafy greens like kale and spinach, fatty fish rich in omega-3 fatty acids, and colorful berries packed with antioxidants are key components. These foods help combat inflammation, a major contributor to endometriosis symptoms.

Gluten and dairy are often identified as inflammatory triggers. The cookbook recommends eliminating or minimizing these from the diet. Gluten-containing grains and dairy products can contribute to inflammation, and their exclusion may provide relief for some individuals.

Maintaining stable blood sugar levels is another crucial aspect. The cookbook suggests incorporating complex carbohydrates, such as whole grains, and lean proteins to prevent blood sugar spikes. Balanced meals help regulate insulin levels, which in turn can positively impact hormonal balance.

Additionally, the cookbook advocates for reducing processed foods and artificial additives. Processed foods often contain trans fats and other chemicals that may exacerbate inflammation. Opting for whole, natural foods supports overall health and the body's ability to manage endometriosis symptoms.

While the Endometriosis Diet Cookbook provides a comprehensive guide, it also encourages individualization. Every person's body reacts differently, and the cookbook acknowledges the need for flexibility in tailoring the diet to personal preferences and tolerances.

In essence, the Endometriosis Diet aims to empower individuals with endometriosis to make informed dietary choices that can positively impact their well-being. Through the incorporation of anti-inflammatory, hormone-balancing, and nutrient-dense foods, the cookbook becomes a valuable tool for managing symptoms and improving the overall quality of life for those navigating the challenges of endometriosis.

ABOUT ENDOMETRIOSIS

Endometriosis is a medical condition where tissue similar to the lining of the uterus, called endometrium, grows outside the uterus. This tissue can be found on the ovaries, fallopian tubes, and other pelvic organs. Endometriosis is a common gynecological disorder that affects people with female reproductive systems, typically during their reproductive years.

Types of Endometriosis

1. Superficial peritoneal endometriosis: The tissue is found on the peritoneum, the thin lining inside the abdomen.

2. Ovarian endometriomas: Cysts formed when endometrial tissue grows on the ovaries.

3. Deep infiltrating endometriosis (DIE): Tissue penetrates more than 5mm below the peritoneum.

Symptoms Of Endometriosis

1. Pelvic pain: Chronic, often accompanied by lower back pain.

2. Painful periods (dysmenorrhea): Severe menstrual cramps.

3. Pain during or after sex (dyspareunia): Especially common during deep penetration.

4. Painful bowel movements or urination: Particularly during menstruation.

5. Excessive bleeding: Heavy or irregular menstrual periods.

6. Infertility: Endometriosis can affect fertility.

Preventive Measures and Management

While there's no surefire way to prevent endometriosis, there are some strategies that may help manage symptoms and improve quality of life:

1. Healthy Diet: Some people find relief through anti-inflammatory diets, as mentioned in the Endometriosis Diet Cookbook.

2. Exercise: Regular physical activity can help manage pain and improve overall well-being.

3. Pain Management: Over-the-counter pain relievers or prescribed medications can alleviate discomfort.

4. Hormonal Therapies: Birth control pills, hormonal IUDs, or other hormonal treatments can help regulate hormones and manage symptoms.

5. Surgery: In severe cases, laparoscopic surgery may be recommended to remove or alleviate endometrial tissue.

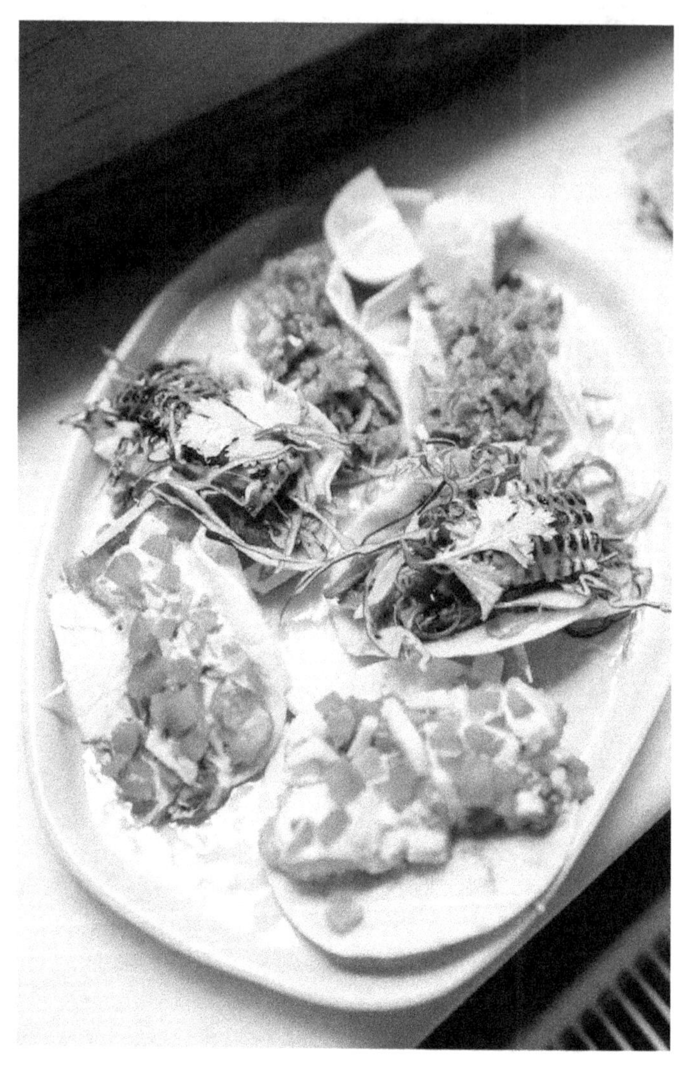

CHAPTER 2: TIPS TO ACHIEVE OPTIMAL HEALTH WITH ENDOMETRIOSIS DIET

The Endometriosis Diet, as recommended by the Endometriosis Diet Cookbook, revolves around selecting foods that promote optimal health while minimizing inflammation and hormonal imbalances associated with endometriosis. This dietary approach aims to manage symptoms and enhance overall well-being.

Foods to Include

1. Leafy Greens: Incorporating a variety of leafy greens such as kale, spinach, and Swiss chard provides essential vitamins and minerals. These greens are rich in antioxidants and anti-inflammatory properties, contributing to overall health and potentially reducing inflammation associated with endometriosis.

2. Fatty Fish: Omega-3 fatty acids found in fish like salmon, mackerel, and sardines can help counter inflammation. These healthy fats may alleviate symptoms and contribute to hormonal balance. Including fish in the diet provides an excellent source of these essential nutrients.

3. Berries: Berries such as blueberries, strawberries, and raspberries are packed with antioxidants. These compounds may help combat oxidative stress and inflammation. Additionally, the natural sweetness of berries can satisfy cravings for sweets without resorting to processed sugars.

4. Whole Grains: Opting for whole grains like quinoa, brown rice, and oats ensures a steady release of energy, stabilizing blood sugar levels. This is crucial in managing hormonal fluctuations that can exacerbate endometriosis symptoms.

5. Lean Proteins: Including lean proteins such as poultry, tofu, and legumes supports muscle health and provides a steady source of energy. Adequate protein intake is essential for overall well-being, especially for individuals managing chronic conditions like endometriosis.

6. Healthy Fats: Incorporating sources of healthy fats, such as avocados, nuts, and olive oil, can contribute to hormonal balance. These fats are essential for the production of hormones and can help alleviate symptoms associated with endometriosis.

7. Colorful Vegetables: A diverse range of vegetables provides an array of nutrients, including vitamins and minerals. Carrots, bell peppers, and sweet potatoes, among others, contribute to a well-rounded, nutrient-rich diet.

Foods to Avoid

1. Gluten: Found in wheat and other grains, gluten can be inflammatory for some individuals. The Endometriosis Diet Cookbook often recommends reducing or eliminating gluten-containing foods like bread and pasta.

2. Dairy: Some individuals with endometriosis find relief by minimizing dairy consumption. Dairy products can contribute to inflammation and hormonal imbalances in certain cases.

3. Processed Foods: Highly processed foods often contain trans fats, additives, and preservatives that may exacerbate inflammation. The cookbook advises against these and encourages a focus on whole, natural foods.

4. Red Meat: While not universally avoided, some individuals with endometriosis choose to limit their intake of red meat due to its potential to contribute to inflammation. Leaner protein sources are often preferred.

5. Caffeine and Alcohol: Excessive consumption of caffeine and alcohol can potentially aggravate endometriosis symptoms. The cookbook may suggest moderating or avoiding these beverages.

6. Highly Sugary Foods: Refined sugars found in candies, pastries, and sugary beverages can lead to blood sugar spikes. Regulating blood sugar is crucial in managing hormonal imbalances, making it advisable to limit these sweet treats.

The Endometriosis Diet Cookbook emphasizes the importance of individualization, acknowledging that each person's body reacts differently to specific foods. It encourages individuals to observe how their bodies respond to different dietary changes and to make adjustments accordingly. Achieving optimum health through an endometriosis diet involves a mindful and personalized approach to nutrition, fostering a strong connection between dietary choices and overall well-being.

CHAPTER 3: BENEFIT OF FOLLOWING ENDOMETRIOSIS DIET

1. Reduced Inflammation: The diet emphasizes anti-inflammatory foods, such as leafy greens, fatty fish, and berries. These can help decrease overall inflammation in the body, potentially alleviating symptoms associated with endometriosis.

2. Hormonal Balance: By including foods that support hormonal balance, such as omega-3 fatty acids from fatty fish and healthy fats from avocados and nuts, the diet aims to manage hormonal fluctuations that can exacerbate endometriosis symptoms.

3. Improved Digestive Health: The focus on whole, nutrient-dense foods and the avoidance of processed foods can contribute to better digestive health. Some individuals with endometriosis experience gastrointestinal symptoms, and a healthy diet can positively impact these issues.

4. Stabilized Blood Sugar Levels: Choosing complex carbohydrates like whole grains helps regulate blood sugar levels. This stability in blood sugar can prevent energy crashes and mood swings, which can be beneficial for those managing endometriosis.

5. Weight Management: A balanced diet that includes lean proteins, healthy fats, and a variety of fruits and vegetables can contribute to weight management. Maintaining a healthy weight is crucial for overall well-being, as excessive weight can contribute to inflammation.

6. Increased Nutrient Intake: The Endometriosis Diet encourages the consumption of a wide variety of nutrient-dense foods, providing essential vitamins and minerals. This can help ensure that individuals with endometriosis are meeting their nutritional needs for overall health.

7. Enhanced Energy Levels: Adopting a diet rich in whole foods and essential nutrients can lead to increased energy levels. This is particularly important for individuals managing chronic conditions like endometriosis, where fatigue is a common symptom.

8. Empowerment and Control: Following the Endometriosis Diet provides individuals with a sense of empowerment and control over their health. Making informed dietary choices based on personal experiences and preferences fosters a proactive approach to managing endometriosis symptoms.

9. Potential Symptom Relief: While individual responses to dietary changes may vary, many individuals report a reduction in endometriosis symptoms, such as pelvic pain, painful periods, and discomfort during intercourse, when following an Endometriosis Diet.

10. Emotional Well-being: A balanced and nourishing diet can positively impact mental and emotional well-being. The sense of control and the physical benefits derived from the diet may contribute to improved mood and reduced stress levels.

CHAPTER 4: HEALTHY RECIPES

LIST OF INGREDIENTS

1. Greek Yogurt:
A rich source of protein and probiotics, beneficial for gut health.

2. Mixed Berries:
Blueberries, strawberries, raspberries - packed with antioxidants that may help reduce inflammation.

3. Granola:
Choose a low-sugar, whole-grain option for added fiber and nutrients.

4. Avocado:
Provides healthy fats and is a good source of vitamin E.

5. Dark Chocolate (70% cocoa):
Contains antioxidants and can be a satisfying treat in moderation.

6. Walnuts:
A source of omega-3 fatty acids and antioxidants.

7. Chia Seeds:
High in fiber and omega-3 fatty acids, beneficial for heart health.

8. Almond Milk:
A dairy-free alternative, rich in vitamin E.

9. Mango:
A tropical fruit providing vitamin C and antioxidants.

10. Vanilla Extract:
Adds flavor without added sugars or artificial sweeteners.

11. Maple Syrup:

A natural sweetener in moderation, avoiding refined sugars.

12. Pineapple Slices:

Contains bromelain, an enzyme with anti-inflammatory properties.

13. Fresh Mint Leaves:

Adds a refreshing flavor and may have digestive benefits.

14. Salmon Fillets:

High in omega-3 fatty acids, known for their anti-inflammatory properties.

15. Quinoa:

A whole grain rich in protein, fiber, and essential minerals.

16. Mixed Vegetables:

Bell peppers, broccoli, carrots - diverse vegetables for a variety of nutrients.

17. Olive Oil:

A heart-healthy oil with anti-inflammatory properties.

18. Garlic:

Contains allicin, known for its potential anti-inflammatory and immune-boosting effects.

19. Fresh Thyme:

An herb with antioxidants and potential anti-inflammatory properties.

20. Fresh Cilantro:

Adds flavor and may have antioxidant and anti-inflammatory benefits.

Berry and Almond Overnight Oats

Ingredients:
- Rolled oats (1/2 cup)
- Almond milk (1/2 cup)
- Greek yogurt (1/4 cup)
- Mixed berries (blueberries, strawberries, raspberries - 1/2 cup)
- Almonds (sliced - 2 tbsp)
- Chia seeds (1 tbsp)
- Honey (1 tbsp)
- Vanilla extract (1/2 tsp)

Instructions:
1. In a jar, combine rolled oats, almond milk, Greek yogurt, mixed berries, sliced almonds, chia seeds, honey, and vanilla extract.
2. Mix well and refrigerate overnight.
3. In the morning, stir the mixture and enjoy a nutrient-packed breakfast.

Spinach and Feta Breakfast Wrap

Ingredients:
- Whole-grain tortilla
- Eggs (2, scrambled)
- Baby spinach (1 cup)
- Feta cheese (2 tbsp, crumbled)
- Cherry tomatoes (1/2 cup, sliced)
- Olive oil (1 tsp)
- Salt and pepper to taste

Instructions:
1. In a pan, sauté baby spinach with olive oil until wilted.
2. Add scrambled eggs and cook until done.
3. Lay out the whole-grain tortilla, and place the spinach and egg mixture on it.
4. Top with crumbled feta and sliced cherry tomatoes.
5. Roll the tortilla into a wrap and enjoy this protein-packed breakfast.

Chia Seed and Mixed Berry Smoothie Bowl

Ingredients:

- Frozen mixed berries (1 cup)
- Almond milk (1/2 cup)
- Greek yogurt (1/4 cup)
- Chia seeds (2 tbsp)
- Honey (1 tbsp)
- Granola (for topping)

Instructions:

1. In a blender, combine frozen berries, almond milk, Greek yogurt, chia seeds, and honey.
2. Blend until smooth and pour into a bowl.
3. Top with granola for added crunch and nutrients.
4. This antioxidant-rich smoothie bowl provides a delicious and nutritious start to the day.

Avocado and Tomato Quinoa Bowl

Ingredients:

- Quinoa (1/2 cup, cooked)
- Avocado (1, sliced)
- Cherry tomatoes (1/2 cup, halved)
- Poached egg (1)
- Fresh cilantro (2 tbsp, chopped)
- Lime juice (1 tbsp)
- Salt and pepper to taste

Instructions:

1. In a bowl, layer cooked quinoa, sliced avocado, and halved cherry tomatoes.
2. Top with a poached egg.
3. Drizzle lime juice over the bowl, sprinkle with fresh cilantro, and season with salt and pepper.
4. A nutrient-dense breakfast that combines healthy fats, protein, and whole grains.

Turmeric and Ginger Infused Smoothie

Ingredients:

- Banana (1, frozen)
- Pineapple chunks (1/2 cup, frozen)
- Greek yogurt (1/2 cup)
- Almond milk (1/2 cup)
- Turmeric powder (1/2 tsp)
- Fresh ginger (1 tsp, grated)
- Chia seeds (1 tbsp)
- Honey (1 tbsp)

Instructions:

1. In a blender, combine frozen banana, pineapple chunks, Greek yogurt, almond milk, turmeric powder, grated ginger, chia seeds, and honey.
2. Blend until smooth and pour into a glass.
3. This anti-inflammatory smoothie provides a refreshing and healthful start to the day.

Quinoa and Roasted Vegetable Salad

Ingredients:
- Quinoa (1 cup, cooked)
- Mixed vegetables (bell peppers, zucchini, cherry tomatoes - 2 cups, chopped)
- Olive oil (2 tbsp)
- Lemon juice (2 tbsp)
- Feta cheese (1/4 cup, crumbled)
- Fresh basil (2 tbsp, chopped)
- Salt and pepper to taste

Instructions:
1. Toss chopped vegetables with olive oil, salt, and pepper.
2. Roast vegetables in the oven until tender.
3. In a bowl, mix cooked quinoa, roasted vegetables, lemon juice, feta cheese, and fresh basil.

4. Serve as a refreshing and nutrient-packed salad.

Lentil and Vegetable Stew

Ingredients:

- Lentils (1 cup, cooked)
- Mixed vegetables (carrots, celery, spinach - 2 cups, chopped)
- Vegetable broth (2 cups)
- Onion (1, diced)
- Garlic (2 cloves, minced)
- Turmeric powder (1/2 tsp)
- Cumin powder (1/2 tsp)
- Olive oil (1 tbsp)
- Salt and pepper to taste

Instructions:

1. Sauté diced onion and minced garlic in olive oil until softened.
2. Add chopped vegetables and cook until slightly tender.
3. Stir in cooked lentils, vegetable broth, turmeric, cumin, salt, and pepper.

4. Simmer until all ingredients are well combined and flavors meld together.
5. A hearty and warming stew with anti-inflammatory ingredients.

Grilled Chicken and Quinoa Bowl

Ingredients:
- Chicken breast (1, grilled and sliced)
- Quinoa (1/2 cup, cooked)
- Broccoli florets (1 cup, steamed)
- Avocado (1, sliced)
- Cherry tomatoes (1/2 cup, halved)
- Lemon vinaigrette (olive oil, lemon juice, Dijon mustard, salt, and pepper)

Instructions:
1. Grill the chicken breast until fully cooked, then slice.
2. In a bowl, arrange cooked quinoa, steamed broccoli, sliced chicken, avocado, and cherry tomatoes.

  3. Drizzle with lemon vinaigrette for a
     light and flavorful lunch.

Chickpea and Spinach Curry

Ingredients:
  - Chickpeas (1 can, drained and rinsed)
  - Fresh spinach (2 cups)
  - Onion (1, diced)
  - Garlic (3 cloves, minced)
  - Coconut milk (1 cup)
  - Curry powder (1 tbsp)
  - Turmeric powder (1/2 tsp)
  - Ginger (1 tsp, grated)
  - Olive oil (1 tbsp)
  - Salt and pepper to taste

Instructions:
  1. Sauté diced onion and minced garlic
     in olive oil until softened.
  2. Add chickpeas, coconut milk, curry
     powder, turmeric, grated ginger, salt,
     and pepper.

3. Simmer until the flavors meld together and the spinach wilts.
4. Serve over brown rice or quinoa for a flavorful and nutritious curry.

Salmon and Asparagus Foil Packets

Ingredients:
- Salmon fillet (1)
- Asparagus spears (1 bunch)
- Lemon slices (2)
- Fresh dill (2 tbsp, chopped)
- Olive oil (2 tbsp)
- Garlic powder (1/2 tsp)
- Salt and pepper to taste

Instructions:
1. Preheat the oven to 400°F (200°C).
2. Place salmon fillet and asparagus on a large piece of foil.
3. Drizzle with olive oil, sprinkle with garlic powder, salt, and pepper.
4. Top with lemon slices and fresh dill.

5. Seal the foil into a packet and bake for 15-20 minutes until salmon is cooked through.

6. A simple and delicious foil packet dinner rich in omega-3 fatty acids.

Mediterranean Chickpea Salad

Ingredients:

- Chickpeas (1 can, drained and rinsed)
- Cucumber (1, diced)
- Cherry tomatoes (1 cup, halved)
- Red onion (1/2, finely chopped)
- Kalamata olives (1/4 cup, sliced)
- Feta cheese (1/4 cup, crumbled)
- Fresh parsley (2 tbsp, chopped)
- Olive oil (2 tbsp)
- Red wine vinegar (1 tbsp)
- Garlic powder (1/2 tsp)
- Oregano (1/2 tsp)
- Salt and pepper to taste

Instructions:

1. In a large bowl, combine chickpeas, cucumber, cherry tomatoes, red onion, olives, and feta cheese.

2. In a small bowl, whisk together olive oil, red wine vinegar, garlic powder, oregano, salt, and pepper.
3. Pour the dressing over the salad and toss well.
4. Serve chilled for a refreshing and satisfying dinner.

Quinoa Stuffed Bell Peppers

Ingredients:

- Bell peppers (4, halved and seeds removed)
- Quinoa (1 cup, cooked)
- Black beans (1/2 cup, cooked and drained)
- Corn kernels (1/2 cup)
- Diced tomatoes (1/2 cup)
- Avocado (1, diced)
- Lime juice (2 tbsp)
- Cumin (1 tsp)
- Chili powder (1/2 tsp)
- Fresh cilantro (2 tbsp, chopped)
- Salt and pepper to taste

Instructions:

1. Preheat the oven to 375°F (190°C).
2. In a bowl, mix cooked quinoa, black beans, corn, diced tomatoes, avocado, lime juice, cumin, chili powder, fresh cilantro, salt, and pepper.
3. Stuff bell peppers with the quinoa mixture.
4. Bake for 25-30 minutes until peppers are tender.
5. A wholesome and colorful dinner option.

Baked Lemon Garlic Salmon with Roasted Vegetables

Ingredients:

- Salmon fillets (2)
- Broccoli florets (2 cups)
- Carrots (1 cup, sliced)
- Lemon (1, sliced)
- Garlic (3 cloves, minced)
- Olive oil (2 tbsp)

- Fresh thyme (1 tbsp, chopped)
- Salt and pepper to taste

Instructions:
1. Preheat the oven to 400°F (200°C).
2. Place salmon fillets on a baking sheet.
3. In a bowl, toss broccoli, carrots, lemon slices, minced garlic, olive oil, fresh thyme, salt, and pepper.
4. Spread the vegetable mixture around the salmon.
5. Bake for 15-20 minutes until the salmon is cooked through and the vegetables are tender.

Eggplant and Chickpea Curry

Ingredients:
- Eggplant (1, diced)
- Chickpeas (1 can, drained and rinsed)
- Coconut milk (1 cup)
- Onion (1, diced)
- Garlic (3 cloves, minced)
- Curry powder (1 tbsp)

- Turmeric powder (1/2 tsp)
- Ginger (1 tsp, grated)
- Olive oil (1 tbsp)
- Fresh cilantro (2 tbsp, chopped)
- Salt and pepper to taste

Instructions:

1. In a pan, sauté diced onion and minced garlic in olive oil until softened.
2. Add diced eggplant and cook until slightly browned.
3. Stir in chickpeas, coconut milk, curry powder, turmeric, grated ginger, salt, and pepper.
4. Simmer until the eggplant is tender.
5. Garnish with fresh cilantro before serving.

Turkey and Vegetable Stir-Fry

Ingredients:

- Ground turkey (1 lb)
- Mixed vegetables (bell peppers, broccoli, snap peas - 2 cups, sliced)
- Soy sauce (3 tbsp)
- Sesame oil (1 tbsp)
- Garlic (2 cloves, minced)
- Ginger (1 tsp, grated)
- Green onions (3, sliced)
- Brown rice (2 cups, cooked)

Instructions:

1. In a wok or large pan, cook ground turkey until browned.
2. Add mixed vegetables, minced garlic, and grated ginger. Stir-fry until vegetables are tender-crisp.

3. In a small bowl, mix soy sauce and sesame oil. Pour over the turkey and vegetables.
4. Stir in sliced green onions.
5. Serve over cooked brown rice for a quick and satisfying dinner.

Berry and Greek Yogurt Parfait

Ingredients:
- Greek yogurt (1 cup)
- Mixed berries (blueberries, strawberries, raspberries - 1 cup)
- Granola (1/2 cup)
- Honey (2 tbsp)
- Mint leaves for garnish

Instructions:
1. In a glass or bowl, layer Greek yogurt, mixed berries, and granola.
2. Drizzle honey over the top.
3. Repeat the layers.
4. Garnish with mint leaves.
5. A delicious and nutritious parfait rich in antioxidants.

Dark Chocolate Avocado Mousse

Ingredients:

- Avocado (2, ripe)
- Dark chocolate (70% cocoa - 1/2 cup, melted)
- Cocoa powder (2 tbsp)
- Maple syrup (1/4 cup)
- Vanilla extract (1 tsp)
- Salt (a pinch)
- Berries for topping

Instructions:

1. In a blender, combine ripe avocados, melted dark chocolate, cocoa powder, maple syrup, vanilla extract, and a pinch of salt.
2. Blend until smooth and creamy.
3. Refrigerate for at least 2 hours.
4. Serve topped with fresh berries.

Baked Apple with Cinnamon and Walnuts

Ingredients:

- Apples (2, cored)
- Cinnamon (1 tsp)
- Walnuts (2 tbsp, chopped)
- Maple syrup (2 tbsp)
- Greek yogurt for serving

Instructions:

1. Preheat the oven to 375°F (190°C).
2. Place cored apples on a baking sheet.
3. In a bowl, mix cinnamon, chopped walnuts, and maple syrup.
4. Stuff each apple with the cinnamon-walnut mixture.
5. Bake for 20-25 minutes or until apples are tender.
6. Serve with a dollop of Greek yogurt.

Chia Seed Pudding with Mango

Ingredients:

- Chia seeds (1/4 cup)
- Almond milk (1 cup)
- Mango (1, diced)
- Vanilla extract (1/2 tsp)
- Maple syrup (1 tbsp)

Instructions:

1. In a jar, mix chia seeds, almond milk, vanilla extract, and maple syrup.
2. Stir well and refrigerate for at least 4 hours or overnight.
3. Before serving, top with diced mango.
4. A satisfying and omega-3 rich chia seed pudding.

Grilled Pineapple with Honey and Mint

Ingredients:

- Pineapple slices (1 cup)
- Honey (2 tbsp)
- Fresh mint leaves (2 tbsp, chopped)
- Greek yogurt for serving

Instructions:

1. Preheat a grill or grill pan.
2. Grill pineapple slices for 2-3 minutes on each side until grill marks appear.
3. Drizzle with honey and sprinkle chopped mint over the top.
4. Serve with a side of Greek yogurt.
5. A simple and refreshing grilled dessert.

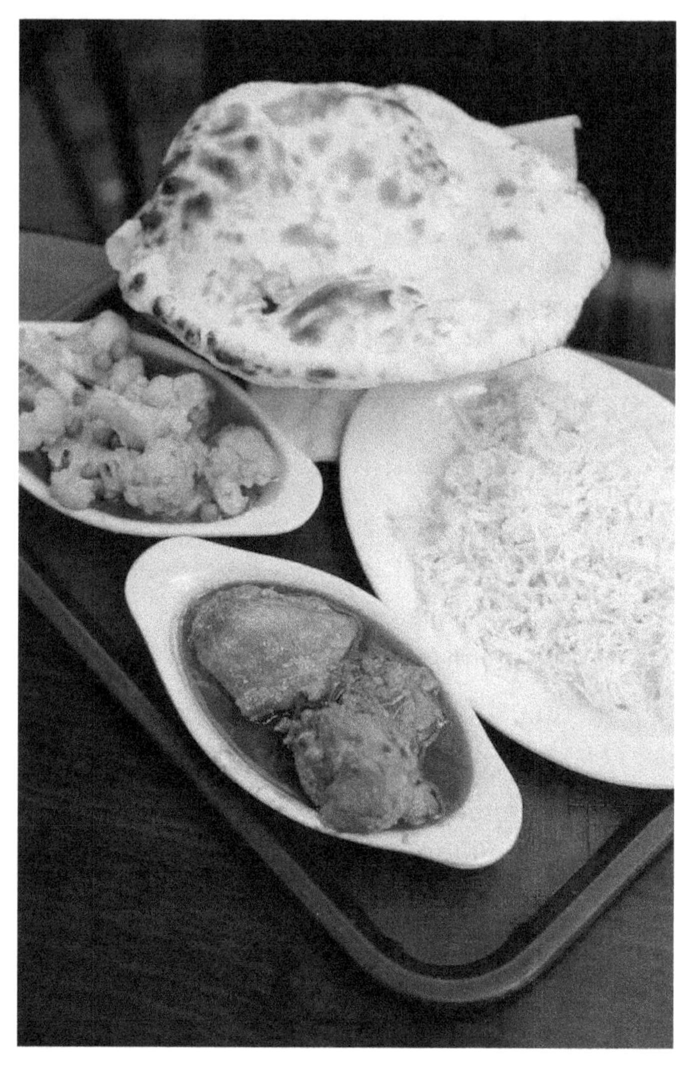

CHAPTER 5: MEAL PLANNING

HOW TO USE THE MEAL PLAN

Review the Meal Plan:

Take a moment to review the entire 14-day meal plan, familiarizing yourself with the variety of recipes and meals scheduled for each day.

Create a Shopping List:

Based on the meal plan, create a shopping list by noting down the ingredients required for each day's breakfast, lunch, and dinner. Ensure you have all the necessary items before starting the week.

Meal Preparation:

Consider batch-cooking certain components or entire meals to save time during the week. For example, you can prepare quinoa, chopped vegetables, or grilled chicken in advance to streamline the cooking process.

Daily Meal Execution:

Follow the meal plan day by day, preparing and enjoying the specified recipes for breakfast, lunch, and dinner. Feel free to make adjustments based on personal taste preferences or dietary restrictions.

Listen to Your Body:

Pay attention to how your body responds to the meals. If there are any ingredients that cause discomfort or if you find certain recipes particularly enjoyable, take note. The meal plan serves as a guide, and personalization is key to its success.

14-DAY MEAL PLAN

Day 1:

Breakfast: Berry and Almond Overnight Oats

Lunch: Quinoa and Roasted Vegetable Salad

Dinner: Grilled Chicken and Quinoa Bowl

Day 2:

Breakfast: Spinach and Feta Breakfast Wrap

Lunch: Lentil and Vegetable Stew

Dinner: Baked Lemon Garlic Salmon with Roasted Vegetables

Day 3:

Breakfast: Chia Seed and Mixed Berry Smoothie Bowl

Lunch: Mediterranean Chickpea Salad

Dinner: Eggplant and Chickpea Curry

Day 4:

Breakfast: Avocado and Tomato Quinoa Bowl

Lunch: Turkey and Vegetable Stir-Fry

Dinner: Salmon and Asparagus Foil Packets

Day 5:

Breakfast: Turmeric and Ginger Infused Smoothie
Lunch: Quinoa Stuffed Bell Peppers
Dinner: Chickpea and Spinach Curry

Day 6:

Breakfast: Dark Chocolate Avocado Mousse
Lunch: Grilled Pineapple with Honey and Mint
Dinner: Quinoa and Roasted Vegetable Salad

Day 7:

Breakfast: Berry and Greek Yogurt Parfait
Lunch: Baked Apple with Cinnamon and Walnuts
Dinner: Baked Lemon Garlic Salmon with Roasted Vegetables

Day 8:

Breakfast: Chia Seed Pudding with Mango
Lunch: Mediterranean Chickpea Salad
Dinner: Eggplant and Chickpea Curry

Day 9:
Breakfast: Vanilla Greek Yogurt with Mixed Berries
Lunch: Turkey and Vegetable Stir-Fry
Dinner: Quinoa Stuffed Bell Peppers

Day 10:
Breakfast: Dark Chocolate Avocado Mousse
Lunch: Lentil and Vegetable Stew
Dinner: Grilled Chicken and Quinoa Bowl

Day 11:
Breakfast: Avocado and Tomato Quinoa Bowl
Lunch: Quinoa and Roasted Vegetable Salad
Dinner: Salmon and Asparagus Foil Packets

Day 12:
Breakfast: Berry and Almond Overnight Oats
Lunch: Chickpea and Spinach Curry
Dinner: Quinoa Stuffed Bell Peppers

Day 13:

Breakfast: Chia Seed Pudding with Mango
Lunch: Spinach and Feta Breakfast Wrap
Dinner: Eggplant and Chickpea Curry

Day 14:

Breakfast: Turmeric and Ginger Infused Smoothie
Lunch: Grilled Pineapple with Honey and Mint
Dinner: Chickpea and Spinach Curry

CONCLUSION

In conclusion, this Endometriosis Diet Cookbook presents a thoughtfully curated collection of recipes designed to align with the principles of an anti-inflammatory diet, potentially aiding those managing endometriosis. By focusing on nutrient-dense ingredients and incorporating a variety of flavors, the cookbook offers a versatile and enjoyable approach to fostering overall well-being.

These recipes not only provide potential relief from symptoms associated with endometriosis but also contribute to enhanced nutritional intake and balanced living. As you embark on this journey, remember that adopting and adapting to this diet is a personal commitment to your health. Empower yourself with the knowledge that small, sustainable changes can yield significant benefits.

Let this cookbook be a guide, offering not just nourishment for the body, but also a path towards holistic wellness. Embrace this journey with determination, and may your commitment to a healthier lifestyle become a source of strength, resilience, and renewed vitality. Your well-being is a priority – you've got this!

Thank you for choosing our Endometriosis Diet Cookbook. We hope these recipes enhance your well-being. Your feedback is invaluable to us – please share your thoughts on the book, its impact, or any improvements we can make. Wishing you health and happiness on your journey to optimal living.

BONUS: WEEKLY MEAL PLANNER JOURNAL

MEAL PLANNER

Weekly

WEEK ______________________   MONTH ______________________

MONDAY

TUESDAY

WEDNESDAY

THURSDAY

FRIDAY

SATURDAY

SUNDAY

SHOPPING LIST

MEAL PLANNER

Weekly

WEEK ___________________ MONTH ___________________

MONDAY

TUESDAY

WEDNESDAY

THURSDAY

FRIDAY

SATURDAY

SUNDAY

SHOPPING LIST

MEAL PLANNER

Weekly

WEEK _______________   MONTH _______________

MONDAY

SATURDAY

TUESDAY

SUNDAY

WEDNESDAY

SHOPPING LIST

THURSDAY

FRIDAY

MEAL PLANNER

Weekly

WEEK _________________________   MONTH _________________________

MONDAY

TUESDAY

WEDNESDAY

THURSDAY

FRIDAY

SATURDAY

SUNDAY

SHOPPING LIST

MEAL PLANNER

Weekly

WEEK ___________________   MONTH ___________________

MONDAY

SATURDAY

TUESDAY

SUNDAY

WEDNESDAY

SHOPPING LIST

THURSDAY

FRIDAY

MEAL PLANNER

Weekly

WEEK __________________________   MONTH __________________________

MONDAY

SATURDAY

TUESDAY

SUNDAY

WEDNESDAY

SHOPPING LIST

THURSDAY

FRIDAY

MEAL PLANNER

Weekly

WEEK ______________________   MONTH ______________________

MONDAY

SATURDAY

TUESDAY

SUNDAY

WEDNESDAY

SHOPPING LIST

THURSDAY

FRIDAY

MEAL PLANNER

Weekly

WEEK __________________________   MONTH __________________________

MONDAY

TUESDAY

WEDNESDAY

THURSDAY

FRIDAY

SATURDAY

SUNDAY

SHOPPING LIST

MEAL PLANNER

Weekly

WEEK ________________   MONTH ________________

MONDAY

TUESDAY

WEDNESDAY

THURSDAY

FRIDAY

SATURDAY

SUNDAY

SHOPPING LIST

-
-
-
-
-
-
-
-
-
-
-
-
-

MEAL PLANNER

Weekly

WEEK ___________________   MONTH ___________________

MONDAY

TUESDAY

WEDNESDAY

THURSDAY

FRIDAY

SATURDAY

SUNDAY

SHOPPING LIST

www.ingramcontent.com/pod-product-compliance
Lightning Source LLC
Chambersburg PA
CBHW050847260726
48660CB00006B/2496